Contents

Contents

1

The Brain's User Manual (That Nobody Gave You)

Let's start with a question: how well do you know your own brain? If you're like most people, the answer is probably "not very well." Despite being the most powerful and complex organ in the human body, your brain didn't exactly come with an instruction manual. The good news? Science has uncovered many of the principles that govern your thoughts, habits, and emotions. By understanding these principles, you can finally start using your brain to your advantage.

In this chapter, we'll cover the basics of how your brain operates, the quirks that can trip you up, and some key concepts that will set the foundation for transforming your mental habits.

1. The Brain's Two Modes: Automatic vs. Deliberate Thinking

Imagine your brain as a car. You have two modes: automatic (cruise control) and deliberate (manual control). Most of the time, your brain operates on autopilot, using established patterns of thought and behavior to save mental energy. This is great when you're brushing your teeth or driving a familiar route. But when faced with complex decisions or unfamiliar challenges, that autopilot can work against you.

This concept is often referred to as **System 1 and System 2 thinking**, a model popularized by psychologist Daniel Kahneman in his book *Thinking, Fast and Slow.*

- **System 1** is fast, emotional, and automatic. It handles instinctual reactions and everyday tasks.
- **System 2** is slow, analytical, and deliberate. It's the system you engage when solving problems or learning new skills.

The trick to mastering your mind is knowing when to switch modes. Too often, people let System 1 dominate situations where careful thought is needed, leading to snap judgments and mistakes. Conversely, some overthink every minor decision, exhausting their mental energy.

2. Neuroplasticity: Rewiring Your Mental Circuits

You might have heard the phrase, "You can't teach an old dog new tricks." Fortunately, that's not true for humans. Your brain has an incredible ability to rewire itself, a concept known as **neuroplasticity**. Every time you learn something new, your brain creates or strengthens neural pathways.

Think of these pathways as hiking trails in the woods. The more you walk down a trail, the clearer and easier it becomes to follow. Similarly, the more you practice a skill or habit, the more ingrained it becomes in your brain.

This is both good and bad news. Good, because it means

you can change habits and learn new things at any age. Bad, because negative patterns—like procrastination, anxiety, or self-doubt—become deeply embedded if left unchecked. The goal is to deliberately create and reinforce positive neural pathways while weakening the negative ones.

3. The Habit Loop: Cue, Routine, Reward

One of the most powerful ways your brain operates is through habits. These automatic routines are governed by a loop with three parts:

1. **Cue** – A trigger that signals the brain to begin a routine.
2. **Routine** – The behavior or action itself.
3. **Reward** – The benefit or relief you gain from completing the routine.

For example, say you have a habit of eating snacks late at night. The cue might be boredom or stress. The routine is grabbing a bag of chips, and the reward is the temporary comfort it provides.

Understanding this loop is the first step to changing habits. If you can identify the cue and reward, you can experiment with different routines that provide similar benefits. Instead of chips, you might try a relaxing activity like reading or stretching to see if it satisfies the same need.

4. Emotional Hijacking: When Your Brain Rebels

Have you ever "lost it" in a moment of frustration, only to regret it later? That's called an **amygdala hijack**—a term coined by psychologist Daniel Goleman. The amygdala, part of the brain's limbic system, is responsible for processing emotions, particularly fear and anger. When you perceive a threat, your amygdala can bypass rational thinking, triggering a fight-or-flight response.

This response was essential for survival in prehistoric times. If you encountered a saber-toothed tiger, you needed to react instantly, not ponder your options. But in the modern world, the "threats" we face are often more psychological—an angry email, a traffic jam, or a critical comment. Unfortunately, your brain doesn't always distinguish between life-or-death emergencies and everyday stressors.

Learning to regulate your emotional responses is crucial. Techniques like deep breathing, grounding exercises, and re-framing negative thoughts can help you regain control when your brain starts to spiral.

5. The Power of Focus and Attention

In a world full of distractions, maintaining focus has become a superpower. Your brain is constantly bombarded with information, and it's easy to get caught in a cycle of multitasking. However, research shows that multitasking reduces productivity by up to 40%. Your brain can only fully focus on one task at a time.

The key to improving focus is **selective attention**—the ability to prioritize what truly matters and block out everything else. Strategies like the **Pomodoro Technique** (working in focused 25-minute intervals) and **time-blocking** (scheduling specific tasks during the day) can help you train your brain to concentrate more effectively.

Additionally, limiting digital distractions, such as turning off notifications and setting screen time limits, can significantly boost your mental clarity.

6. Cognitive Biases: Your Brain's Built-In Shortcuts

Your brain loves shortcuts, which are often helpful but can also lead to irrational decisions. These mental shortcuts, known as **cognitive biases**, influence how you perceive the world. Here are a few common examples:

- **Confirmation bias**: The tendency to seek out information that confirms your existing beliefs.
- **Negativity bias**: Giving more weight to negative experiences than positive ones.
- **Anchoring bias**: Relying too heavily on the first piece of information you encounter.

By becoming aware of these biases, you can challenge your assumptions and make more rational decisions.

7. Putting It All Together

Now that you understand the basics of how your brain works, you have a foundation for transformation. Throughout the rest of this book, we'll explore practical strategies to harness your brain's full potential. You'll learn how to change negative thought patterns, build new habits, and stay focused in a chaotic world.

Remember: your brain is an incredible tool. But like any tool, it requires maintenance and practice to use it effectively. The more you understand and work with your mind, the more control you'll gain over your life.

2

Automatic Negative Thoughts (ANTs) and How to Crush Them

You're standing in line at the coffee shop when a thought suddenly pops into your head: *Why did I say that in the meeting? Everyone probably thinks I'm a fool.* You replay the scenario over and over, scrutinizing every word and imagining the worst-case scenario. That, my friend, is an automatic negative thought—or **ANT**—at work.

ANTs are spontaneous, pessimistic thoughts that creep into your mind without invitation. They tend to be irrational and self-defeating but can feel incredibly real and overwhelming in the moment. The good news? You don't have to let them take over your mental space. In this chapter, we'll explore why ANTs occur, how to recognize them, and effective strategies to crush them before they crush you.

1. What Are Automatic Negative Thoughts (ANTs)?

ANTs are the mental equivalent of weeds in a garden. Just as weeds can sprout without warning, negative thoughts can infiltrate your mind, often fueled by fear, anxiety, or self-doubt. They tend to be reactive and automatic, arising in response to specific situations or triggers.

Here are some common examples:

- *I'm not good enough to do this job.*
- *Everyone is judging me.*
- *This will never work out.*
- These thoughts often stem from cognitive distortions—biased ways of thinking that skew our perception of reality.

2. Cognitive Distortions: The Root of ANTs

Cognitive distortions are mental traps that lead to negative thinking. Psychologist Aaron Beck, a pioneer of cognitive therapy, identified several common distortions that fuel ANTs. Let's break down a few of the most common ones:

- **All-or-Nothing Thinking**: Viewing situations in extremes, such as "I'm either a success or a failure."
- **Catastrophizing**: Expecting the worst possible outcome, even when the likelihood is low.
- **Mind Reading**: Assuming you know what others are thinking (and assuming it's negative).
- **Overgeneralization**: Believing that one negative event is part of a never-ending pattern of failure.
- **Personalization**: Taking responsibility for events outside of your control, e.g., "It's my fault they're upset."

Recognizing these distortions is the first step in breaking the cycle of automatic negative thoughts.

3. Why Does Your Brain Default to Negativity?

Our brains are wired to prioritize negative information—a phenomenon known as the **negativity bias**. This bias evolved to keep our ancestors alert to danger. Back then, missing a sign of danger could mean death, so our brains developed a tendency to focus on threats.

In the modern world, this survival mechanism works against us. Instead of lions and tigers, we worry about deadlines, social rejection, and financial stress. The brain still treats these modern stressors as life-or-death situations, amplifying negative thoughts.

Understanding that this bias is natural—and not necessarily a reflection of reality—can help you put your thoughts in perspective.

4. Identifying Your Triggers

Certain situations are more likely to trigger ANTs. These triggers are often linked to past experiences, fears, or insecurities. For example, someone who experienced frequent criticism in childhood might be prone to negative self-talk whenever they receive feedback at work.

Take some time to reflect on situations that tend to bring out your ANTs. Common triggers include:

· High-pressure situations (e.g., public speaking)
· Social interactions
· Conflict or criticism

- Uncertainty about the future

Once you identify your triggers, you can anticipate when negative thoughts are likely to arise and prepare to counteract them.

5. Challenging Negative Thoughts

The next step in defeating ANTs is to challenge them. Here's a simple but effective process called **thought disputation**:

1. **Identify the thought**: Write down the negative thought as soon as you notice it.
2. **Examine the evidence**: Ask yourself, "What evidence supports this thought? What evidence contradicts it?"
3. **Consider alternative perspectives**: What would you say to a friend who had this thought? Can you think of a more balanced or neutral viewpoint?
4. **Replace the thought**: Create a new thought that is more rational and empowering. For example, replace "I always mess things up" with "I made a mistake, but I can learn from it."

By consistently practicing this technique, you'll start to weaken the power of negative thoughts.

6. Reframing: Turning Negatives into Positives

Reframing is a powerful mental shift that allows you to view challenges in a more constructive light. Instead of focusing on what's wrong, you focus on what you can learn or gain from the situation.

For example, imagine you didn't get a promotion at work. An automatic negative thought might be, *I'm a failure.* Through reframing, you could tell yourself, *This is an opportunity to improve my skills and be even more prepared next time.*

Reframing doesn't mean ignoring negative emotions. It's about acknowledging them while choosing to focus on growth and possibilities.

7. The Power of Gratitude

Gratitude is the antidote to negativity. Research shows that practicing gratitude can rewire your brain to focus more on positive experiences. When you regularly reflect on what you're thankful for, you create new neural pathways that counterbalance the brain's negativity bias.

Here are a few simple ways to incorporate gratitude into your routine:

- **Gratitude journaling**: Write down three things you're grateful for each day.
- **Gratitude meditation**: Spend a few minutes reflecting on positive moments or people in your life.
- **Expressing gratitude**: Tell someone you appreciate them, whether through a text, call, or handwritten note.

Over time, these practices can help shift your mental focus away from automatic negativity.

8. The Role of Self-Compassion

Self-compassion is another key tool in combating ANTs. Instead of beating yourself up for having negative thoughts, treat yourself with kindness and understanding. According to psychologist Dr. Kristin Neff, self-compassion involves three components:

- **Self-kindness**: Offering yourself the same empathy you would give a friend.
- **Common humanity**: Recognizing that everyone experiences challenges and negative thoughts.
- **Mindfulness**: Being aware of your thoughts and feelings without judgment.

Practicing self-compassion can reduce the intensity of ANTs and help you build emotional resilience.

9. Creating Mental Space with Mindfulness

Mindfulness involves observing your thoughts without getting caught up in them. By cultivating mindfulness, you can create mental space between yourself and your negative thoughts, allowing you to respond rather than react.

Try this simple mindfulness exercise:

1. Sit quietly and focus on your breath.
2. When a negative thought arises, label it (e.g., "That's worry" or "That's fear").
3. Gently bring your attention back to your breath without judgment.

With regular practice, mindfulness can help you become more aware of your thought patterns and less reactive to negativity.

10. Building a Positive Thought Routine

Finally, develop a daily routine to reinforce positive thinking. This might include:

- **Morning affirmations**: Start your day with empowering statements.
- **Daily reflection**: Spend a few minutes reflecting on positive moments at the end of each day.
- **Visualization**: Imagine yourself succeeding in future challenges to build confidence.

By consistently practicing these techniques, you'll strengthen the positive neural pathways in your brain, making it easier to stay optimistic and resilient.

In the next chapter, we'll explore how stress and overthinking keep you trapped in negative thought loops—and how to break free for good.

3

Why You Can't Stop Thinking About Work (Even on Vacation)

You finally made it. After months of back-to-back meetings and endless emails, you're on vacation, sitting by the pool with a cold drink in hand. But instead of enjoying the moment, your mind drifts back to work: *Did I forget to send that report? What if something goes wrong while I'm gone?*

Sound familiar? You're not alone. Many people find it difficult to disconnect from work, even during their downtime. In this chapter, we'll explore why this happens, how chronic work stress affects your brain, and practical strategies to help you truly switch off and recharge.

1. The Science of Overthinking

Overthinking is a mental habit where your brain gets stuck in repetitive thought loops. Psychologists call this process **rumination**. When you ruminate, you repeatedly analyze problems, potential outcomes, and perceived threats—often without reaching any solutions. This mental cycle can be exhausting and counterproductive.

So, why does your brain do this? It's largely due to your **stress response system**, also known as the "fight-or-flight" mechanism. When you're under stress, your brain's **amygdala** (the emotional processing center) kicks into high gear, sending signals to stay alert. This response is meant to protect you from danger, but in today's world, your brain interprets emails, deadlines, and performance reviews as threats.

Because modern work environments are filled with constant stressors, your brain becomes conditioned to stay on high alert, even during your personal time.

2. The Role of Cortisol and Stress Hormones

When you're stressed, your body releases **cortisol**, a hormone designed to help you react to threats. In short bursts, cortisol is helpful. It increases focus and energy, giving you the ability to tackle challenges. However, chronic stress causes your cortisol levels to remain elevated, which can lead to:

- Poor concentration
- Difficulty relaxing or falling asleep
- Increased anxiety
- Physical symptoms like headaches and muscle tension

Over time, this state of heightened alertness can trap you in a cycle of overthinking and burnout. Even when you're supposed to be relaxing, your brain struggles to "turn off" because it's still on the lookout for potential work-related problems.

3. The Perfectionism Trap

For many people, perfectionism is a major contributor to work-related rumination. If you hold yourself to impossibly high standards, you're more likely to dwell on your mistakes, replay conversations, and worry about being judged by colleagues or supervisors.

Common perfectionist thoughts include:

· *I can't afford to make any mistakes.*
· *If I'm not constantly on top of things, I'll fall behind.*
· *Others are expecting me to be perfect.*

This mindset creates a constant state of pressure, making it difficult to relax and delegate tasks, even when you're out of the office.

4. The Myth of Hustle Culture

Society often glorifies **hustle culture**—the idea that constant productivity is the key to success. You've probably heard phrases like:

· *"Sleep is for the weak."*
· *"Grind now, rest later."*
· *"If you're not working, someone else is outworking you."*

These messages reinforce the belief that taking breaks or vacations is a sign of laziness or lack of ambition. Over time, this mindset can erode your ability to prioritize rest, leading to chronic overwork and diminished performance.

The reality is that rest is essential for peak productivity. Numerous studies have shown that regular breaks and vacations improve creativity, problem-solving skills, and overall well-being. In other words, working yourself to exhaustion doesn't make you more successful—it makes you less effective.

5. Setting Boundaries with Technology

One of the biggest barriers to disconnecting from work is the **always-on culture** enabled by technology. Thanks to smartphones, email notifications, and collaboration apps, it's easier than ever to stay connected to work 24/7.

Here's a common scenario: You receive an email marked "urgent" after hours. Even if you don't respond immediately, your mind starts racing with possible solutions. This one notification pulls you out of relaxation mode and back into work mode.

To break this cycle, you need to establish boundaries with your devices. Try the following strategies:

- **Turn off notifications** during non-work hours.
- **Set email boundaries** by letting colleagues know when you're unavailable.
- **Create a tech-free zone** at home, such as your bedroom or dining area.

By reducing your exposure to work-related notifications, you give your brain the chance to fully relax.

6. The Art of Detachment Rituals

A **detachment ritual** is an intentional practice that signals to your brain that it's time to switch from work mode to relaxation mode. These rituals can be simple but powerful in helping you mentally disconnect.

Examples include:

- **A daily shutdown routine**: At the end of each workday, spend 10 minutes organizing your tasks for the next day and saying, "Work is done for now."
- **Physical movement**: Exercise, stretch, or take a walk to transition out of your work mindset.
- **Mindful breathing**: Spend a few minutes focusing on your breath to center yourself and release tension.

These rituals create a psychological boundary between your work life and personal life, helping you avoid the trap of endless overthinking.

7. Delegating and Trusting Others

If you're struggling to disconnect from work, ask yourself: **Am I trying to do everything myself?** Many people who experience work-related anxiety have difficulty delegating tasks because they fear others won't meet their standards.

However, trying to manage everything on your own is unsustainable. Delegation is not just about offloading tasks—it's about trusting your team and empowering them to take ownership of their responsibilities. When you delegate effectively, you reduce your mental load and give yourself permission to focus on other areas of your life.

8. The Role of Self-Compassion

Work-related stress often stems from being overly critical of yourself. If you catch yourself ruminating on mistakes or perceived shortcomings, try practicing **self-compassion**. Remind yourself that:

- Everyone makes mistakes.
- Perfection is not required to succeed.
- You are doing your best in a challenging environment.

Treat yourself with the same kindness and understanding you would offer a friend. This shift in mindset can help reduce the intensity of negative thoughts and ease your transition into relaxation mode.

9. Practicing Mental "Vacations"

Even when you're not on a physical vacation, you can give your mind a break by practicing **mental vacations**. This involves engaging in activities that fully absorb your attention and provide a sense of joy or relaxation.
Examples include:

- Immersing yourself in a creative hobby, like painting or writing
- Spending time in nature
- Playing games or puzzles that challenge your brain in fun ways

By regularly scheduling mental breaks, you train your brain to step away from work-related concerns and recharge more effectively.

10. Redefining Success

Finally, take a step back and reflect on your definition of success. Is it tied solely to your work achievements? If so, you may be placing too much pressure on yourself to constantly perform. Consider expanding your definition of success to include areas like:

- Personal growth and learning
- Relationships and community involvement
- Physical and mental health

By shifting your focus to a more holistic view of success, you can reduce the anxiety and overthinking that keeps you trapped in work mode.

In the next chapter, we'll dive into the importance of creating space for pause and reflection, and how this practice can help you avoid emotional overreactions.

4

The Power of Pause: Training Yourself to Stop Overreacting

Have you ever snapped at someone in the heat of the moment and immediately regretted it? Or found yourself paralyzed by anxiety, unable to think clearly? These are examples of emotional reactions hijacking your brain. The good news is that you can retrain your mind to pause before you react—giving yourself time to choose a more measured response.

In this chapter, we'll explore why your brain reacts so strongly to stress, how to recognize when you're being emotionally hijacked, and practical techniques to build a pause into your reactions. This skill can improve your relationships, decision-making, and overall mental well-being.

1. Understanding Emotional Hijacking

When you experience a sudden surge of fear, anger, or anxiety, your **amygdala**—the brain's emotional center—takes control. This is known as an **amygdala hijack**, a term coined by psychologist Daniel Goleman in his book *Emotional Intelligence*.

The amygdala perceives threats and triggers a fight-or-flight response designed to protect you from danger.

The problem is that in today's world, many of these "threats" aren't actually life-threatening. A harsh email, an argument with a colleague, or a missed deadline can set off your amygdala just as a predator would have in prehistoric times. When this happens, your **prefrontal cortex**—the part of your brain responsible for rational thinking—gets overridden.

This is why you might say or do things in the heat of the moment that you wouldn't normally consider wise.

2. The Consequences of Reacting Without a Pause

Reacting impulsively can have negative consequences, including:

- **Damaged relationships**: Heated words or aggressive behavior can strain personal and professional connections.
- **Regret**: You might replay the situation later and wish you had handled it differently.
- **Increased stress**: Emotional outbursts can leave you feeling drained and ashamed, perpetuating anxiety.
- **Poor decisions**: When emotions cloud your judgment, you may make choices that don't serve your long-term goals.

Learning to pause before reacting helps you maintain control, allowing your rational mind to catch up and assess the situation.

3. Recognizing the Signs of an Emotional Hijack

The first step to managing emotional reactions is to recognize when you're being hijacked by your emotions. Common physical and mental signs include:

- Rapid heart rate
- Tension in your muscles (especially the neck, shoulders, and jaw)
- Shallow breathing or holding your breath
- Racing thoughts or difficulty concentrating
- A strong urge to react immediately (e.g., yelling, sending an angry email)

When you notice these signs, it's a signal to pause and engage in calming techniques.

4. The Power of the 3-Second Rule

A simple but effective technique to avoid overreacting is the **3-second rule**. When you feel triggered, pause for three seconds before responding. In those few seconds, you can take a deep breath and ask yourself:

- Is this reaction going to help or hurt the situation?
- What outcome do I want from this interaction?
- How can I express myself in a way that aligns with my values?

This brief pause allows your prefrontal cortex to regain control, giving you the clarity to choose a more thoughtful response.

5. Deep Breathing: A Quick Reset Tool

One of the fastest ways to calm your nervous system is through **deep breathing**. When you're stressed, your breathing becomes shallow and rapid, signaling to your brain that you're in danger. By intentionally slowing your breath, you can send a message to your brain that you are safe.

Try this simple breathing exercise:

1. Inhale slowly through your nose for a count of four.
2. Hold your breath for a count of four.
3. Exhale slowly through your mouth for a count of six.
4. Repeat this cycle three to five times.

This practice activates your **parasympathetic nervous system**, which helps reduce the fight-or-flight response.

6. Reframing the Situation

Reframing involves looking at a situation from a different perspective. Often, our emotional reactions are based on assumptions rather than facts. By reframing, you can challenge those assumptions and reduce your emotional intensity.

For example, imagine you receive a blunt email from a coworker. Your initial thought might be, *They're being rude and disrespectful.* However, by pausing and reframing, you might consider alternative explanations, such as *Maybe they were in a hurry or under pressure.*

Reframing helps you stay curious rather than reactive, which can prevent misunderstandings and unnecessary conflict.

7. Grounding Techniques to Stay Present

When your mind spirals into anxiety or anger, grounding techniques can bring you back to the present moment. These techniques anchor your attention to your physical surroundings, helping you regain control of your thoughts and emotions.

Here are a few grounding exercises to try:

- **5-4-3-2-1 technique**: Identify five things you can see, four things you can touch, three things you can hear, two things you can smell, and one thing you can taste.
- **Body scan**: Focus on each part of your body, starting from your toes and moving upward, noticing any tension and consciously relaxing each area.
- **Sensory focus**: Hold a small object (like a pen or key) and concentrate on its texture, temperature, and weight.

These techniques can quickly interrupt emotional overwhelm and help you stay calm.

8. The Role of Emotional Regulation

Emotional regulation is the ability to manage your emotional responses in a way that aligns with your goals and values. It doesn't mean suppressing or ignoring your emotions—it means acknowledging them without letting them control your actions.

Here are some strategies to build emotional regulation:

- **Name your emotions**: Simply labeling what you're feeling (e.g., "I'm frustrated") can reduce its intensity.
- **Practice self-compassion**: Remind yourself that it's normal to feel strong emotions and that you're doing your best.
- **Use positive self-talk**: Replace negative thoughts with

affirmations, such as *I can handle this calmly.*

With regular practice, these techniques can help you become more emotionally resilient.

9. The Importance of Self-Awareness

Developing self-awareness is key to mastering the power of pause. By understanding your emotional triggers and patterns, you can anticipate situations where you're likely to overreact and prepare strategies in advance.

Start by reflecting on recent emotional incidents. Ask yourself:

- What triggered my reaction?
- How did I feel physically and emotionally in the moment?
- What thoughts went through my mind?
- How could I have responded differently?

Over time, this reflection process will help you build greater control over your responses.

10. Practicing the Pause in Everyday Life

The pause is a skill that improves with practice. You don't have to wait for high-stakes situations to practice it. Try integrating pauses into your daily routine:

- **Before responding to texts or emails**: Take a few moments to think about your message.
- **During conversations**: Pause briefly before speaking to

ensure your response is thoughtful.
- **At the end of the day**: Reflect on moments where you paused and how it impacted your interactions.

The more you practice, the more natural it will become to pause and respond rather than react impulsively.

Mastering the power of pause can transform your relationships, reduce stress, and improve your decision-making. In the next chapter, we'll explore how your inner critic sabotages your success—and how to finally silence it for good.

5

Your Inner Critic Is Fired

Have you ever heard a voice in your head saying things like, *You're not smart enough for this,* or *Why do you always mess things up?* That voice is your **inner critic**—a relentless commentator that thrives on self-doubt, fear, and negativity. It often masquerades as helpful by pushing you to do better, but in reality, it's a major saboteur of confidence and success.

The inner critic isn't a permanent resident in your mind. You can learn to challenge, quiet, and even transform it into a more constructive inner voice. In this chapter, we'll explore where the inner critic comes from, how it affects your mindset and performance, and strategies to fire it once and for all.

1. What Is the Inner Critic?

The inner critic is a mental narrative that focuses on your perceived flaws, mistakes, and shortcomings. It often disguises itself as self-improvement advice but tends to be overly harsh and unforgiving. Psychologists refer to this voice as a form of **negative self-talk**, and it can take various forms, including:

- **Perfectionism**: "You'll never be good enough unless you do everything perfectly."
- **Catastrophizing**: "If you fail, everyone will see you as a failure forever."
- **Imposter syndrome**: "You don't deserve to be here. Sooner or later, people will figure out you're a fraud."

These thoughts can feel automatic and unshakeable, but they are not reflections of reality. They are mental habits that have developed over time.

2. Where Does the Inner Critic Come From?

The inner critic is often shaped by early life experiences. It may have originated from:

- **Critical authority figures**: Parents, teachers, or mentors who frequently pointed out your mistakes.
- **Peer pressure and social comparison**: Experiences of being judged, excluded, or ridiculed can create self-critical thought patterns.
- **Perfectionist environments**: Growing up in an environment that valued high achievement may have instilled a belief that you're only worthy if you perform flawlessly.

Your brain internalizes these messages and creates a self-monitoring system to avoid future criticism or rejection. While this mechanism might have helped you stay "safe" in the past, it now holds you back from growth and confidence.

3. How the Inner Critic Affects Your Life

The inner critic impacts various areas of your life, often without you realizing it. Here's how it can manifest:

- **Procrastination**: You delay tasks because you fear they won't be perfect.
- **Low self-esteem**: You believe you're not capable or deserving of success.
- **Overwork and burnout**: You push yourself too hard to avoid perceived failure.
- **Social anxiety**: You worry excessively about being judged or rejected.

These patterns reinforce each other, creating a cycle of self-sabotage. Breaking the cycle requires identifying and challenging the critic's narrative.

4. Recognizing Your Inner Critic's Voice

To quiet your inner critic, you first need to recognize when it's speaking. Pay attention to your self-talk in moments of stress or failure. Common phrases might include:

- "I'm such an idiot."
- "They probably think I'm incompetent."
- "Why do I always mess up?"

Once you become aware of these thoughts, you can start to separate yourself from them. Remember: **You are not your thoughts.** The inner critic is just one voice in your mind—not the truth.

5. Challenging Negative Self-Talk

The next step is to challenge your inner critic with evidence and logic. Here's how:

1. **Identify the thought**: Write down the negative thought your inner critic is repeating.
2. **Examine the evidence**: Ask yourself, "Is this thought 100% true?" Often, you'll realize it's based on assumptions rather than facts.
3. **Consider alternative perspectives**: What would a supportive friend say about this situation?
4. **Create a balanced response**: Replace the negative thought with a more realistic and compassionate statement.

For example, if your inner critic says, *You're a failure because you made a mistake,* you could reframe it as, *Everyone makes mistakes. This is an opportunity to learn and improve.*

6. Replacing the Critic with a Coach

Instead of letting your inner critic dominate your thoughts, cultivate an inner **coach**—a voice that is encouraging, compassionate, and solution-focused. Your inner coach helps you learn from challenges without tearing you down.

Here's an example of how the two voices differ:

- **Inner Critic**: "You'll never get this right. Why even try?"
- **Inner Coach**: "This is tough, but you've handled challenges before. Let's break it down step by step."

Practice speaking to yourself in the same way you would support a friend. Over time, your inner coach will become stronger and more natural.

7. Practicing Self-Compassion

Self-compassion is the antidote to the inner critic. According to Dr. Kristin Neff, self-compassion involves three components:

- **Self-kindness**: Treating yourself with empathy and understanding, especially during difficult moments.
- **Common humanity**: Recognizing that everyone experiences struggles and setbacks.
- **Mindfulness**: Being aware of your thoughts and feelings without judgment or over-identification.

By practicing self-compassion, you create a mental environment where growth and resilience can thrive.

8. The Power of Positive Affirmations

Positive affirmations can help rewire your brain to focus on your strengths rather than your shortcomings. These are short, empowering statements that counteract negative self-talk. Examples include:

- "I am capable and worthy of success."
- "I can handle challenges with grace and confidence."
- "I learn and grow from my experiences."

Repeat these affirmations daily, especially during moments of doubt. Over time, they can become a natural part of your thought process.

9. Avoiding Perfectionism Traps

Perfectionism fuels the inner critic by setting impossible standards. To break free from perfectionism, remind yourself that:

- **Done is better than perfect**: Completing a task is more valuable than obsessing over every detail.
- **Mistakes are opportunities to learn**: Failure is a normal part of growth and innovation.
- **You are enough**: Your worth is not tied to your achievements.

Set realistic goals and celebrate progress rather than perfection.

10. Building a Support System

You don't have to face your inner critic alone. Surround yourself with supportive people who encourage and uplift you. Share your struggles with trusted friends, mentors, or a therapist who can offer perspective and advice.

Hearing external validation and encouragement can help you internalize a more positive self-image.

11. Rewriting Your Narrative

Your inner critic often clings to outdated narratives about who you are and what you're capable of. To overcome this, start rewriting your personal story. Reflect on:

- Your strengths and accomplishments
- Challenges you've overcome
- Moments where you surprised yourself with your resilience

By focusing on your growth and potential, you can reshape your self-identity in a more empowering way.

12. Moving Forward Without the Critic

Firing your inner critic doesn't mean you'll never experience self-doubt again. However, it does mean you'll have the tools to manage it. By practicing self-compassion, positive self-talk, and emotional resilience, you can quiet the voice that once held you back and step into your full potential.

In the next chapter, we'll explore how to transform anxiety into a source of motivation and energy.

6

How to Turn Anxiety into Motivation

Anxiety has a bad reputation. It's often seen as something to be avoided at all costs—a sign of weakness or a barrier to success. But what if I told you that anxiety doesn't have to be the enemy? In fact, when managed correctly, it can become a powerful motivator. Anxiety is simply energy. The key is learning how to channel that energy in a way that fuels your goals rather than derails them.

In this chapter, we'll explore how anxiety works, the difference between harmful and helpful anxiety, and practical strategies to transform it into motivation and productivity.

1. What Is Anxiety, Really?

Anxiety is your body's natural response to perceived threats. It activates your **sympathetic nervous system**, releasing stress hormones like adrenaline and cortisol to prepare you for action. This response is commonly known as **fight-or-flight**.

Anxiety becomes a problem when your brain perceives everyday challenges—such as a presentation, deadline, or social event—as life-threatening. This overreaction triggers physical symptoms such as:

- Racing heart
- Shallow breathing
- Sweating or trembling
- Restlessness and racing thoughts

However, anxiety can also be helpful in small doses. It sharpens your focus, heightens your senses, and motivates you to take action. The key is learning to regulate the intensity so that it works *for* you rather than against you.

2. The Yerkes-Dodson Law: Finding Your Optimal Stress Zone

You may not realize it, but some anxiety is essential for peak performance. This idea is captured by the **Yerkes-Dodson law**, which suggests that performance improves with increased arousal (or stress) up to a certain point. Beyond that point, too much anxiety causes performance to decline.

Imagine an inverted U-shaped curve:

- **Low arousal (too little anxiety)**: You feel bored, unfocused, and unmotivated.
- **Optimal arousal (moderate anxiety)**: You're energized, alert, and fully engaged in the task.
- **High arousal (too much anxiety)**: You feel overwhelmed, panicked, and unable to concentrate.

The goal is to stay in the "sweet spot" of optimal arousal, where anxiety enhances your performance without overpowering you.

3. Identifying Helpful vs. Harmful Anxiety

Not all anxiety is created equal. **Helpful anxiety** serves a purpose—it alerts you to important tasks and motivates you to prepare. For example:

- Feeling nervous before a job interview may push you to practice your answers and research the company.
- Worrying about a deadline may encourage you to prioritize your work and stay focused.

On the other hand, **harmful anxiety** can paralyze you with fear and prevent you from taking action. It often involves worst-case scenario thinking, such as:

- *If I fail this presentation, my entire career is over.*
- *Everyone will think I'm a complete failure.*

The key is learning to harness helpful anxiety while managing harmful anxiety.

4. Reframing Anxiety as Excitement

One powerful technique for managing anxiety is **reframing** it as excitement. Physiologically, anxiety and excitement are nearly identical—they both increase your heart rate, adrenaline, and alertness. The difference lies in your mindset.

The next time you feel anxious about a challenge, try telling yourself, "I'm excited." For example:

- Instead of *I'm anxious about this presentation*, say *I'm excited*

37

to share my ideas.
- Instead of *I'm nervous about this test,* say *I'm excited to show what I've learned.*

This simple mental shift can reduce your fear and boost your confidence.

5. Channeling Anxiety into Action

Anxiety often arises from uncertainty and lack of control. By taking proactive steps, you can regain a sense of control and reduce your anxiety. Here's how:

1. **Break tasks into smaller steps**: Overwhelming projects can trigger anxiety. Break them down into manageable tasks and focus on one step at a time.
2. **Create a plan**: Outline what needs to be done, set deadlines, and prioritize tasks. This helps reduce ambiguity and gives you a clear roadmap.
3. **Take immediate action**: Even a small step forward can shift your mindset from *frozen* to *focused.* For example, if you're anxious about an exam, start by reviewing one chapter.

Action interrupts the anxiety cycle and builds momentum.

6. Practicing "Productive Worry"

Productive worry involves using your anxiety to identify potential challenges and create solutions in advance. It's different from **unproductive worry**, which involves endless rumination without any action.

Here's how to practice productive worry:

1. **Write down your concerns**: List the specific things you're anxious about.
2. **Identify possible solutions**: For each concern, brainstorm practical steps you can take to address it.
3. **Focus on what you can control**: Let go of worries about things outside your control and concentrate on actionable items.

By turning your worries into a plan, you can reduce uncertainty and feel more prepared.

7. Using Visualization to Build Confidence

Visualization is a mental exercise where you imagine yourself succeeding in a challenging situation. This technique helps condition your brain to associate the task with positive outcomes rather than fear.

Try this visualization exercise:

1. Close your eyes and take a few deep breaths.
2. Picture yourself in the situation that makes you anxious (e.g., giving a presentation).
3. Imagine yourself performing confidently and calmly. Visualize everything going well, including your body language, tone of voice, and reactions from others.
4. Repeat this exercise daily leading up to the event.

Visualization can reprogram your brain to expect success rather than failure.

8. The Role of Physical Activity

Physical activity is one of the most effective ways to manage anxiety. Exercise releases endorphins—your body's natural stress relievers—and helps burn off excess adrenaline.

Incorporate movement into your daily routine with activities such as:

- Walking or jogging
- Yoga or stretching
- Strength training or sports

Even short bursts of activity, like a 10-minute walk, can have a significant impact on your mood and energy levels.

9. Practicing Self-Compassion During Anxiety

When anxiety strikes, it's easy to be hard on yourself. You might think, *I should be able to handle this better.* However, self-criticism only amplifies anxiety.

Instead, practice **self-compassion** by reminding yourself:

- Anxiety is a normal part of life.
- You're doing your best in a challenging situation.
- You deserve kindness and patience.

By treating yourself with empathy, you create a mental environment that supports growth and resilience.

10. Building Resilience Through Reflection

After facing an anxiety-inducing challenge, take time to reflect on what you learned. Ask yourself:

- What went well?
- What could I improve next time?
- How did I manage my anxiety during the situation?

Reflection helps you build emotional resilience by reinforcing positive behaviors and identifying areas for growth. Over time, you'll develop greater confidence in your ability to handle anxiety.

11. Creating an Anxiety Management Toolkit

To turn anxiety into motivation, build a personal toolkit of strategies that work for you. This might include:

- Deep breathing exercises
- Positive affirmations
- Visualization techniques
- Physical activity
- Support from friends, mentors, or a therapist

Experiment with different approaches and refine your toolkit as needed.

12. Moving Forward with Anxiety as Your Ally

Anxiety doesn't have to be an obstacle. When channeled effectively, it can become a source of energy, focus, and motivation. By learning to regulate your anxiety and harness its power, you can achieve greater success and resilience in all areas of your life.

In the next chapter, we'll explore how multitasking might be sabotaging your productivity—and whether there's a way to make it work for you. Stay tuned!

7

Mindful Multitasking: Myth or Magic?

You're answering emails while listening to a podcast and making notes for an upcoming meeting. You feel productive, but by the end of the day, you can't remember much of what you did. Sound familiar? Multitasking has become the norm in today's fast-paced world, but research shows that it's not as efficient as we think.

In this chapter, we'll examine the myth of multitasking, its impact on your brain, and whether there's a mindful approach that can help you manage multiple tasks without losing focus or efficiency.

1. The Multitasking Myth

Many people believe that multitasking—juggling multiple tasks at once—makes them more productive. However, studies have repeatedly shown that the brain is not designed to focus on more than one cognitively demanding task at a time. What we think of as multitasking is actually **task-switching**, where the brain rapidly shifts attention between tasks.

Each time you switch tasks, your brain experiences a **cognitive load**—the mental effort required to refocus. This can lead to:

- **Reduced efficiency**: Task-switching slows you down, as your brain takes time to "reload" the information needed for each task.
- **Increased errors**: Splitting your attention increases the likelihood of mistakes.
- **Mental fatigue**: Constant task-switching can exhaust your brain, leaving you feeling scattered and drained.

2. The Cost of Multitasking on Your Brain

Multitasking can have a range of negative effects on your mental performance, including:

- **Short-term memory overload**: Your working memory has limited capacity. When you try to juggle multiple tasks, you overload this system, making it harder to retain information.
- **Reduced focus**: Frequent interruptions prevent deep focus, reducing your ability to complete complex or creative tasks.
- **Stress and anxiety**: The constant pressure to manage multiple tasks can activate your stress response, increasing cortisol levels and anxiety.

In the long term, habitual multitasking can impair your ability to concentrate, even when you're trying to focus on just one task.

3. When Multitasking Might Work

Although multitasking is generally inefficient, there are situations where it can be effective. These include:

- **Combining a physical and mental task**: For example, you might listen to a podcast while exercising. Because exercise doesn't require significant cognitive effort, your brain can focus on the podcast.
- **Routine, automatic tasks**: If you're doing a mindless activity, like folding laundry, you can multitask by mentally engaging in another task, such as brainstorming ideas.

The key is to avoid multitasking when both tasks require your full attention.

4. The Power of Single-Tasking

Single-tasking—focusing on one task at a time—is the antidote to the chaos of multitasking. When you single-task, you give your full attention to the task at hand, which can lead to:

- **Increased productivity**: You complete tasks more quickly and accurately.
- **Deeper focus**: Concentrating on one task allows you to enter a state of flow, where you're fully immersed and highly productive.
- **Reduced stress**: Focusing on one thing at a time can create a sense of control and calm.

The challenge is resisting the urge to check your phone, emails, or other distractions that pull you away from deep work.

5. Practicing Mindful Multitasking

While single-tasking is ideal for complex tasks, there are ways to engage in **mindful multitasking** for less demanding situations. Mindful multitasking involves being fully present and intentional about how you allocate your attention.

Here's how to do it:

1. **Identify tasks that can be combined**: For example, you might listen to a training video while walking on a treadmill.
2. **Set a clear intention**: Decide which task is your primary focus. For example, if you're exercising while listening to a podcast, prioritize listening.
3. **Avoid switching tasks mid-stream**: Once you've chosen your tasks, stick with them until completion. Avoid interruptions like checking messages or switching to other activities.

Mindful multitasking helps you stay grounded and prevents the mental fatigue associated with constant task-switching.

6. Creating a Focus-First Environment

Your environment plays a crucial role in your ability to focus. To reduce distractions and improve concentration, try these strategies:

- **Designate a workspace**: Set up a dedicated area for work or study that's free from distractions.

- **Eliminate digital interruptions**: Turn off notifications on your phone and computer. Use apps like Focus@Will or Freedom to block distracting websites.
- **Use noise management**: If you're sensitive to noise, consider using noise-canceling headphones or listening to white noise to create a calming atmosphere.

Creating a focus-friendly environment sets the stage for productive single-tasking or mindful multitasking.

7. Time-Blocking: A Strategy for Deep Work

Time-blocking is a productivity technique that involves scheduling specific blocks of time for focused work on a single task. By dedicating uninterrupted time to each task, you can avoid the pitfalls of multitasking.

Here's how to implement time-blocking:

1. **Identify your top priorities**: Choose two or three key tasks to focus on for the day.
2. **Schedule blocks of time**: Allocate 60- to 90-minute blocks for each task. Include short breaks between blocks to recharge.
3. **Protect your time**: Treat these blocks as non-negotiable appointments. Let colleagues know you're unavailable during these periods.

Time-blocking helps you maintain focus and create a rhythm for deep, sustained work.

8. The Pomodoro Technique for Sustained Focus

The **Pomodoro Technique** is a time management method designed to enhance focus and prevent burnout. It involves breaking your work into short, focused intervals (typically 25 minutes), followed by a brief break.

Here's how it works:

1. **Set a timer** for 25 minutes.
2. **Work on a single task** without distractions.
3. **Take a 5-minute break** when the timer goes off.
4. **Repeat the cycle** four times, then take a longer break (15-30 minutes).

This technique trains your brain to concentrate in manageable bursts and prevents mental fatigue.

9. Managing Interruptions and Distractions

Interruptions are a major obstacle to productivity. To minimize them:

- **Set boundaries**: Communicate with coworkers and family about your focus times.
- **Use a "do not disturb" signal**: Place a sign or indicator on your desk to signal when you're in deep work mode.
- **Batch tasks**: Group similar tasks (e.g., checking emails, returning calls) and handle them during specific time slots rather than throughout the day.

By proactively managing interruptions, you can maintain momentum and focus.

10. Training Your Brain for Focus

Focus is a skill that can be developed with practice. Try these exercises to improve your concentration:

- **Mindfulness meditation**: Spend 5-10 minutes each day focusing on your breath. When your mind wanders, gently bring your attention back to your breath.
- **Visualization**: Before starting a task, visualize yourself completing it successfully and staying focused.
- **Brain games**: Engage in activities that require sustained attention, such as puzzles, chess, or memory games.

With consistent practice, you'll strengthen your brain's ability to stay focused and resist distractions.

11. Letting Go of Multitasking Guilt

It's easy to feel guilty when you're not doing "all the things" at once. However, true productivity isn't about doing more—it's about doing what matters most. Give yourself permission to focus fully on one task at a time and trust that this approach will yield better results in the long run.

12. Moving Forward with Clarity and Focus

By understanding the limitations of multitasking and embracing mindful work strategies, you can achieve greater productivity, focus, and well-being. In the next chapter, we'll explore how to build habits that stick, even when motivation is low. Stay tuned!

8

Habits That Stick (Even When You Don't Want Them To)

You've probably heard the phrase, "Motivation gets you started, but habits keep you going." It's true. While motivation can be powerful, it's also fleeting. Habits, on the other hand, are your brain's autopilot system. Once established, they can keep you moving forward—even on days when you don't feel like it. But how do you build habits that last?

In this chapter, we'll explore the science behind habit formation, common reasons why habits fail, and proven strategies to create habits that stick.

1. The Habit Loop: Cue, Routine, Reward

The foundation of every habit is a **loop** with three key components:

1. **Cue**: A trigger that prompts the behavior.
2. **Routine:** The behavior or action itself.
3. **Reward**: A benefit or sense of satisfaction that reinforces

the behavior.

For example, if you have a habit of checking your phone first thing in the morning, the habit loop might look like this:

- **Cue**: Waking up
- **Routine**: Grabbing your phone and scrolling through social media
- **Reward**: Dopamine hit from new notifications and updates

Understanding this loop is crucial because it helps you identify which part of the habit needs to change. By modifying the cue, routine, or reward, you can break bad habits and create new ones.

2. Why Good Habits Are Hard to Build (and Bad Habits Are Hard to Break)

Good habits often require effort and delayed gratification, while bad habits provide instant rewards. For example, eating a donut feels good right away, but the long-term consequences (e.g., weight gain) are delayed. In contrast, exercising requires effort up front, and the rewards—better health, improved mood—come later.

This difference in timing makes bad habits easier to form and good habits harder to maintain. However, by designing your environment and reward system strategically, you can overcome these challenges.

3. Start Small: The Power of Micro-Habits

One of the biggest mistakes people make is trying to change too much too quickly. You might set ambitious goals like going to the gym every day, only to burn out after a week. Instead, focus on **micro-habits**—small, easy actions that are almost impossible to fail at.

Examples of micro-habits include:

- Doing one push-up each morning
- Meditating for one minute
- Writing one sentence in a journal

These tiny actions build momentum and confidence, making it easier to expand the habit over time.

4. Habit Stacking: Building on Existing Routines

Habit stacking involves linking a new habit to an existing one. This technique leverages the fact that your brain is already accustomed to certain routines. By anchoring new habits to these routines, you increase the likelihood of success.

Here's how it works:

1. Identify an existing habit (e.g., brushing your teeth).
2. Add a new habit right after or before it (e.g., doing five squats).
3. Repeat the sequence consistently until it becomes automatic.

An example habit stack might look like this:

- *After I pour my morning coffee, I will write down three things*

I'm grateful for.

5. Focus on Identity, Not Outcomes

Many people set habits based on outcomes (e.g., losing weight, writing a book), but these goals can feel overwhelming and distant. Instead, focus on building an identity. Ask yourself, **"Who do I want to become?"**

For example, instead of saying, "I want to lose 20 pounds," frame your habit as, "I am someone who makes healthy choices." By aligning your habits with your desired identity, you reinforce positive behaviors through self-image.

6. Use Immediate Rewards to Reinforce Good Habits

One of the reasons bad habits stick is that they provide immediate gratification. To build good habits, you need to create **short-term rewards** that motivate you in the moment.

Here are some ways to reward yourself:

- **Gamify your progress**: Track your streaks and celebrate milestones.
- **Pair a habit with something enjoyable**: Listen to your favorite podcast while exercising.
- **Use positive reinforcement**: After completing a habit, say something encouraging to yourself, like *"Great job!"*

Over time, the intrinsic benefits of the habit (e.g., improved health, increased confidence) will take over as the primary motivator.

7. Design Your Environment for Success

Your environment plays a crucial role in shaping your habits. If your surroundings are filled with temptations and distractions, it's harder to stick to positive routines. Conversely, a well-designed environment can make good habits easier to maintain.

Here are some tips to optimize your environment:

- **Make good habits convenient**: Place workout clothes by your bed if you want to exercise in the morning.
- **Remove temptations**: Keep junk food out of sight if you're trying to eat healthier.
- **Create visual cues**: Use reminders, sticky notes, or habit trackers to prompt action.

Small changes in your environment can have a significant impact on your behavior.

8. Anticipate and Overcome Obstacles

Even the best intentions can be derailed by unexpected challenges. By anticipating obstacles in advance, you can develop strategies to stay on track.

Common obstacles include:

- **Lack of time**: Plan habits into your schedule and prioritize them like appointments.
- **Low motivation**: Remind yourself of your "why" and focus on small wins to build momentum.
- **Setbacks**: Accept that setbacks are normal and not a sign of failure. Use them as learning opportunities.

Creating an "if-then" plan can help you navigate obstacles. For example, *"If I can't make it to the gym, I'll do a 10-minute workout at home."*

9. Accountability and Social Support

Having an accountability partner or support system can significantly increase your chances of success. Share your goals with someone you trust and check in regularly to discuss your progress.

You can also join groups or communities with similar goals. The sense of belonging and encouragement can keep you motivated when your willpower wanes.

10. Habit Tracking: Visualizing Your Progress

Tracking your habits provides a sense of accomplishment and keeps you motivated. Use a journal, app, or habit tracker to monitor your progress. Each time you complete a habit, check it off your list.

The visual reminder of your progress creates a positive reinforcement loop. Over time, you'll develop a streak that you won't want to break—a phenomenon known as the **"don't break the chain"** method, famously used by comedian Jerry Seinfeld to maintain his writing habit.

11. Be Patient: Habits Take Time

It's a common misconception that habits form in 21 days. In reality, research suggests it takes an average of **66 days** to establish a habit, depending on the complexity of the behavior.

Some habits may take even longer.

The key is to stay consistent and be patient with yourself. Focus on progress, not perfection, and trust that small actions will compound over time.

12. Building a System for Long-Term Success

Habits are most effective when they're part of a larger system. Instead of relying on willpower alone, create routines and structures that support your goals.

For example, if your goal is to write a book, your system might include:

- **Daily writing sessions** (even if only for 10 minutes)
- **Accountability check-ins** with a writing group
- **Weekly progress reviews** to track milestones

A well-designed system keeps you moving forward, even when motivation fades.

By implementing these strategies, you can create habits that stick—habits that become automatic, sustainable, and aligned with your long-term goals. In the next chapter, we'll explore how to build resilience and bounce back from setbacks.

9

Rewiring for Resilience: The Brain's Bounce-Back Effect

Life is full of setbacks, challenges, and unexpected obstacles. Resilience—the ability to bounce back from adversity—isn't just something people are born with. It's a skill that can be developed, and your brain plays a crucial role in building it. Thanks to **neuroplasticity**, your brain has the capacity to adapt and grow stronger in the face of difficulty.

In this chapter, we'll explore how resilience works at the brain level, how to shift your mindset to embrace challenges, and practical strategies to cultivate mental toughness.

1. What Is Resilience?

Resilience is the ability to recover from setbacks, adapt to change, and keep moving forward in the face of challenges. It doesn't mean avoiding or denying pain and failure. Instead, resilient people acknowledge their difficulties but refuse to be defined by them.

Resilience has several key components:

- **Emotional regulation**: Staying calm and managing your emotions under pressure.
- **Optimism**: Believing that you can overcome challenges and that setbacks are temporary.
- **Problem-solving**: Taking proactive steps to find solutions rather than dwelling on problems.
- **Adaptability**: Adjusting your plans and expectations when circumstances change.

By strengthening these components, you build a mental foundation for handling life's ups and downs.

2. Neuroplasticity: Your Brain's Secret Weapon

Your brain is not static. It has the ability to rewire itself based on your experiences and behaviors—a concept known as **neuroplasticity**. Each time you face a challenge and respond with resilience, you create and strengthen neural pathways that support adaptive thinking.

For example, when you overcome fear in a high-pressure situation, your brain learns to associate that situation with courage rather than panic. Over time, these experiences create a "resilience circuit" in your brain, making it easier to handle future challenges.

The key to leveraging neuroplasticity is **repetition and reflection**. The more you practice resilient behaviors, the more ingrained they become in your mind.

3. The Growth Mindset: Embracing Challenges

Psychologist Carol Dweck introduced the concept of the **growth**

mindset—the belief that abilities and intelligence can be developed through effort, learning, and persistence. In contrast, a **fixed mindset** assumes that talents and abilities are static and unchangeable.

A growth mindset is essential for resilience because it reframes setbacks as opportunities for growth rather than signs of failure. People with a growth mindset are more likely to:

- Persevere through difficulties
- Learn from mistakes
- Seek out feedback and new strategies

To cultivate a growth mindset, practice telling yourself:

- *I can learn from this.*
- *Failure is part of the process.*
- *With effort, I can improve.*

4. The Role of Self-Talk in Resilience

Your **inner dialogue**—the thoughts you tell yourself—can either strengthen or weaken your resilience. Negative self-talk, such as *I can't handle this* or *I always mess up,* reinforces feelings of helplessness. On the other hand, positive and constructive self-talk helps you stay focused and motivated.

Here are some examples of resilience-boosting self-talk:

- *I've overcome tough situations before, and I can do it again.*
- *This is a challenge, not a catastrophe.*
- *What's one small step I can take right now?*

By becoming aware of your self-talk and intentionally shifting it, you can build a more resilient mindset.

5. Reframing Setbacks as Opportunities

One of the most powerful tools for resilience is **reframing**—the ability to view a situation from a different, more constructive perspective. For example, instead of seeing a failed project as a personal failure, you can reframe it as a learning experience that will help you improve in the future.

To practice reframing, ask yourself:

- What can I learn from this situation?
- How might this challenge help me grow?
- What strengths have I developed through past difficulties?

Reframing doesn't mean ignoring negative emotions. It's about acknowledging your feelings while choosing to focus on growth and possibilities.

6. Building Emotional Regulation Skills

Resilience requires the ability to manage your emotions, especially in stressful situations. Emotional regulation involves recognizing your feelings without being overwhelmed by them. Techniques such as **deep breathing** and **grounding exercises** can help you stay calm and centered.

Here's a simple emotional regulation exercise:

1. **Pause** and take a deep breath when you feel overwhelmed.

2. **Acknowledge** your emotions by labeling them (e.g., "I'm feeling anxious").
3. **Focus** on your breath or a calming mantra, such as *"I am in control."*

Practicing these techniques regularly can help you respond to challenges with greater composure.

7. The Power of Social Support

Resilience is not a solo endeavor. Having a strong support system can make a significant difference in how you cope with adversity. Supportive relationships provide:

- **Emotional comfort**: A safe space to express your feelings and receive empathy.
- **Practical advice**: Guidance and problem-solving ideas from people you trust.
- **Encouragement**: Reminders of your strengths and capabilities.

Reach out to friends, family, mentors, or colleagues when you face challenges. Don't be afraid to ask for help—it's a sign of strength, not weakness.

8. Developing a Resilience Routine

Resilience isn't just about reacting to crises. It's about building daily habits that strengthen your mental and emotional well-being. Consider incorporating the following practices into your routine:

- **Gratitude journaling**: Write down three things you're grateful for each day.
- **Mindfulness meditation**: Spend 5-10 minutes focusing on your breath to center your mind.
- **Exercise**: Physical activity helps reduce stress and improve mood.
- **Sleep hygiene**: Prioritize rest to recharge your mind and body.

These habits create a foundation of resilience that helps you handle challenges with greater ease.

9. Learning from Resilient Role Models

Look to people who have demonstrated resilience in their lives. This could include historical figures, mentors, or even friends and family members. Study how they overcame obstacles, adapted to setbacks, and maintained hope in difficult circumstances.

Ask yourself:

- What strategies did they use to stay resilient?
- How can I apply those strategies in my own life?
- What qualities do I admire about their mindset?

Learning from others can inspire you to develop your own resilience toolkit.

10. Tracking Your Progress and Growth

Resilience is a skill that grows over time. Regularly reflect on your progress by asking:

- How have I handled challenges differently in the past few months?
- What new strengths have I developed?
- What setbacks have I learned from?

Celebrate your progress, no matter how small. Recognizing your growth reinforces your belief in your ability to overcome future obstacles.

11. The Importance of Self-Compassion

Being resilient doesn't mean being tough all the time. It's important to show yourself compassion during difficult moments. Remind yourself that it's okay to feel vulnerable or uncertain. Self-compassion helps you stay motivated and reduces the risk of burnout.

Practice self-compassion by:

- Speaking to yourself with kindness
- Allowing yourself to rest and recover
- Acknowledging that struggles are a normal part of life

12. Moving Forward with Resilience

Resilience is not about avoiding adversity—it's about facing it head-on and coming out stronger. By developing a growth mindset, building supportive habits, and embracing challenges, you can train your brain to bounce back from setbacks and thrive in the face of uncertainty.

In the next chapter, we'll explore how to manage emotional overwhelm in frustrating situations and prevent minor annoyances from ruining your day.

10

When Everything Annoys You: Emotional Regulation Hacks

We've all been there. Your alarm doesn't go off, someone cuts you off in traffic, and you spill coffee on your shirt. By mid-morning, even the smallest inconveniences—like a colleague's loud typing or an empty printer—can push you over the edge. When life feels overwhelming, your brain can get stuck in a heightened emotional state, where frustration and irritability take control.

In this chapter, we'll explore why minor annoyances can have such a big impact on your mood, how emotional escalation works, and practical hacks to regulate your emotions and regain control over your day.

1. Why Do Small Annoyances Feel So Big?

When you're already under stress, your brain's ability to handle additional frustrations weakens. This is known as **emotional flooding**, where your emotional response system becomes overloaded. The brain interprets small annoyances as larger threats, amplifying your irritation.

Key contributors to emotional flooding include:

- **Chronic stress**: When stress hormones like cortisol remain elevated, your tolerance for frustration decreases.
- **Fatigue**: Lack of sleep impairs emotional regulation, making you more reactive.
- **Accumulated frustrations**: A series of small setbacks can build up and trigger an outburst.

Recognizing these patterns is the first step in breaking the cycle of irritability.

2. The Role of the Amygdala in Emotional Reactions

The **amygdala**, your brain's emotional processing center, is responsible for detecting threats and initiating the fight-or-flight response. When you encounter a stressor—big or small—the amygdala reacts before your rational mind has a chance to intervene.

This can lead to disproportionate emotional reactions, such as yelling at a coworker over a minor issue. To regulate your emotions, you need to engage the **prefrontal cortex**, the part of your brain responsible for reasoning and decision-making. Techniques like deep breathing and reframing can help calm the amygdala and restore balance.

3. The Power of the "Pause Button"

When you feel your frustration rising, one of the most effective tools is the **pause button**—a deliberate moment of stillness before reacting. This pause gives your brain time to shift from emotional reactivity to rational thinking.

Try this exercise:

1. **Take a deep breath**: Inhale slowly through your nose for four seconds, hold for four seconds, and exhale for six seconds.
2. **Acknowledge your emotion**: Label what you're feeling (e.g., "I'm frustrated because of the delay").
3. **Choose your response**: Ask yourself, "What's the best way to handle this situation?"

Even a brief pause can prevent impulsive reactions and help you respond thoughtfully.

4. Reframing Annoyances

Reframing involves changing the way you interpret a situation. Often, annoyances are exacerbated by the stories we tell ourselves. For example, if someone cuts you off in traffic, you might think, *That driver is disrespectful!* This thought increases your anger. However, if you reframe it as, *Maybe they're rushing to an emergency,* your frustration decreases.

Ask yourself:

- Is there another way to look at this situation?
- What assumptions am I making?
- How would I feel if I gave the other person the benefit of the doubt?

Reframing helps you break the cycle of negative thinking and reduce emotional intensity.

5. The Five-Second Rule for Irritation

When you're about to react to an annoyance, try counting backward from five. This simple technique, popularized by Mel Robbins, interrupts your brain's automatic reaction and creates a moment of awareness.

Here's how it works:

1. When you feel triggered, silently count down: **5, 4, 3, 2, 1**.
2. Redirect your focus to a calming action, such as deep breathing or repeating a positive mantra.
3. Proceed with a measured response.

This technique helps you shift from impulsive reactions to deliberate action.

6. Grounding Techniques for Instant Calm

When you're overwhelmed, grounding techniques can help anchor you in the present moment. These techniques use your senses to break the cycle of rumination and emotional escalation.

Try the **5-4-3-2-1 technique**:

- **5**: Identify five things you can see.
- **4**: Identify four things you can touch.
- **3**: Identify three things you can hear.

- **2**: Identify two things you can smell.
- **1**: Identify one thing you can taste.

This exercise shifts your attention away from your frustration and back to your immediate surroundings.

7. Understanding Your Emotional Triggers

Certain situations or behaviors may trigger stronger emotional reactions than others. These triggers often stem from past experiences, insecurities, or unmet needs.
   Take some time to reflect on your triggers:

- What situations tend to irritate you the most?
- What underlying beliefs or fears might be driving your reactions?
- How can you prepare for these situations in the future?

By increasing your self-awareness, you can anticipate triggers and develop strategies to stay calm.

8. The Power of Humor

Humor is a powerful tool for diffusing tension and shifting your emotional state. Finding something to laugh about—even in frustrating situations—can reduce stress and help you regain perspective.

Try these strategies:

- **Look for the absurd**: Ask yourself, *Will this be funny later?*

Sometimes recognizing the absurdity of a situation can lighten your mood.

- **Watch or read something funny**: A quick break to watch a comedy clip or read a funny article can lift your spirits.
- **Laugh at yourself**: Self-deprecating humor can help you take yourself less seriously.

Laughter triggers the release of endorphins, which improve your mood and reduce stress.

9. Resetting Your Mood with a Quick Break

Sometimes, the best way to manage frustration is to step away from the situation. Taking a short break allows your brain to reset and prevents emotional escalation.

Effective break activities include:

- **Taking a walk**: Physical movement helps release pent-up tension.
- **Listening to calming music**: Music can influence your emotional state and promote relaxation.
- **Practicing deep breathing or meditation**: Even a few minutes of mindfulness can restore balance.

By giving yourself time to reset, you can return to the situation with a clearer mind.

10. Practicing Gratitude to Shift Your Focus

When you're stuck in a cycle of frustration, gratitude can help shift your perspective. Research shows that gratitude reduces

stress, improves mood, and enhances overall well-being.
Here's a simple gratitude exercise:

1. Write down three things you're grateful for.
2. Reflect on why these things matter to you.
3. Take a moment to appreciate the positive aspects of your
   life.

This practice trains your brain to focus on what's going right,
rather than fixating on annoyances.

11. Managing Your Energy Levels

Your ability to regulate emotions is closely tied to your physical
energy levels. When you're tired, hungry, or dehydrated, you're
more prone to irritability. Take care of your body by:

- Getting enough sleep
- Eating balanced meals and staying hydrated
- Taking regular breaks to recharge

Maintaining your energy levels helps you stay resilient in the
face of daily frustrations.

12. Developing a Daily Calm Practice

To build long-term emotional resilience, incorporate calming
practices into your daily routine. These might include:

- **Morning meditation** to set a positive tone for the day
- **Evening reflection** to process and release any built-up

    tension
- **Mindful breathing** throughout the day to stay grounded

Consistent practice helps you build a buffer against stress, making it easier to handle life's annoyances with grace.

By applying these emotional regulation hacks, you can prevent small irritations from snowballing into major stressors. In the next chapter, we'll explore quick and effective mental resets that you can use to regain focus and clarity throughout your day.

11

The Daily Mind Reset: 5-Minute Practices for Clarity and Focus

We all have days where life feels overwhelming, with a constant stream of distractions, responsibilities, and emotional stressors competing for our attention. When your mind is cluttered, productivity suffers, and you may feel stuck in a fog. That's where a **mind reset** comes in—a quick, intentional practice to clear your thoughts, regain focus, and boost your mental energy.

In this chapter, we'll explore a variety of 5-minute resets designed to help you recharge throughout your day. These techniques are simple yet powerful ways to break the cycle of stress, overthinking, and distraction.

1. What Is a Mind Reset and Why Do You Need It?

A mind reset is like hitting the mental "refresh" button. Just as your computer slows down when too many programs are running, your brain can become overwhelmed by competing thoughts and tasks. A short break to clear your mind can restore cognitive function, improve focus, and increase emotional balance.

Mind resets are particularly useful during:

- **Transitions** (e.g., between meetings or tasks)
- **Stressful moments** when you feel anxious or overwhelmed
- **Periods of mental fatigue** when concentration wanes

The goal is not to eliminate all thoughts but to create mental space for clarity and focus.

2. The 5-5-5 Breathing Technique

This simple breathing exercise helps calm your nervous system and reduce anxiety. It's perfect for moments of high stress or mental overload.

Here's how it works:

1. **Inhale** slowly through your nose for a count of 5 seconds.
2. **Hold** your breath for 5 seconds.
3. **Exhale** slowly through your mouth for 5 seconds.
4. Repeat the cycle for 2-3 minutes.

This practice activates your **parasympathetic nervous system**, which counteracts the fight-or-flight response and promotes relaxation.

3. The 5-Minute Brain Dump

When your mind is racing with thoughts, tasks, and worries, a **brain dump** can help you offload mental clutter. This exercise involves writing down everything on your mind without filtering or organizing.

Steps:

1. Set a timer for 5 minutes.
2. Write down every thought, task, and concern that comes to mind.
3. Once the timer goes off, review your list and identify actionable items.

This process helps you declutter your mind, prioritize tasks, and let go of non-urgent worries.

4. Visualization for Mental Clarity

Visualization is a powerful tool to reset your mind and refocus on your goals. By mentally rehearsing success, you create positive neural pathways that enhance motivation and confidence.

Try this quick visualization exercise:

1. Close your eyes and take a few deep breaths.
2. Visualize yourself completing a task with ease and confidence.
3. Imagine the positive feelings you'll experience once the task is done.
4. Open your eyes and approach the task with renewed focus.

This practice can boost your performance by priming your brain for success.

5. Grounding with the 5-4-3-2-1 Technique

Grounding techniques help anchor your mind in the present moment, breaking the cycle of rumination and anxiety. The **5-4-3-2-1 technique** uses your senses to shift your focus.

Steps:

1. Identify **5** things you can see.
2. Identify **4** things you can touch.
3. Identify **3** things you can hear.
4. Identify **2** things you can smell.
5. Identify **1** thing you can taste.

This exercise helps you reconnect with your surroundings and regain a sense of calm.

6. Micro-Meditation

You don't need 30 minutes to benefit from meditation. A **micro-meditation** can provide a quick mental reset in just a few minutes.
Steps:

1. Find a quiet spot and sit comfortably.
2. Close your eyes and focus on your breath.
3. When your mind wanders, gently bring your attention back to your breath.
4. Continue for 2-5 minutes.

Regular micro-meditation can improve concentration, emotional regulation, and resilience over time.

7. The Gratitude Reset

Gratitude shifts your focus from what's wrong to what's going right, which can immediately improve your mood and perspective.

Steps:

1. Take a few moments to reflect on three things you're grateful for.
2. Write them down or say them aloud.
3. Focus on why these things matter to you and how they enhance your life.

This practice rewires your brain to notice and appreciate positive experiences, reducing stress and negativity.

8. Physical Movement Breaks

Your mind and body are deeply connected. Physical movement can help reset your brain by releasing tension and boosting endorphins.

Try one of these quick movement exercises:

- **Stretching**: Focus on your neck, shoulders, and back—areas that hold tension.
- **Walking**: Take a short walk, even if it's just around your office or home.
- **Quick workout**: Do 5-10 push-ups, squats, or jumping jacks to increase blood flow.

Even a few minutes of movement can improve focus and energy.

9. Repeating Positive Affirmations

Positive affirmations help replace negative self-talk with empowering beliefs. This practice is especially useful when you're feeling doubtful or overwhelmed.

Steps:

1. Choose a positive statement, such as *"I am capable and confident"* or *"I can handle whatever comes my way."*
2. Repeat the affirmation silently or aloud for 2-5 minutes.
3. Focus on the feeling of confidence and empowerment that the words evoke.

Affirmations reinforce a resilient mindset and encourage positive behavior.

10. Digital Detox: A 5-Minute Tech Break

Constant notifications and screen time can overload your brain. Taking short tech breaks can help reduce mental fatigue and restore focus.

Steps:

1. Turn off your phone or put it in "do not disturb" mode.
2. Step away from your computer or other devices.
3. Spend 5 minutes doing a non-digital activity, such as stretching, journaling, or simply sitting quietly.

Regular tech breaks improve your ability to concentrate and reduce digital burnout.

11. Progressive Muscle Relaxation

Progressive muscle relaxation (PMR) helps release physical tension, which often accumulates during stressful situations. Steps:

1. Start with your feet. Tense the muscles for a few seconds, then release.
2. Move upward through your body, tensing and relaxing each muscle group (legs, stomach, arms, shoulders, jaw).
3. Focus on the sensation of relaxation as you release tension.

This exercise promotes deep relaxation and can reset both your mind and body.

12. Building a Daily Reset Routine

The key to maintaining mental clarity and focus is consistency. Consider scheduling regular mind resets throughout your day, such as:

- **Morning reset**: Set intentions and visualize a successful day.
- **Midday reset**: Take a movement or breathing break to recharge.
- **Evening reset**: Reflect on your accomplishments and practice gratitude.

These routines create a foundation for sustained mental well-being and productivity.

By incorporating these 5-minute practices into your day, you can stay calm, focused, and energized, even in the face of stress and distractions. In the next and final chapter, we'll develop a personalized mental playbook to help you win at life.

12

Winning at Life: A Mental Playbook

You've explored how your mind works, learned strategies to manage your thoughts and emotions, and built habits that strengthen your resilience and productivity. Now, it's time to put everything together into a personal **mental playbook**—a set of strategies and practices that you can rely on to navigate life's challenges, stay focused on your goals, and live with purpose and clarity.

In this chapter, we'll create a step-by-step guide to maintaining mental well-being, setting achievable goals, and continuously growing in both your personal and professional life.

1. Defining What "Winning" Means to You

Success looks different for everyone. Before you can build a plan for your life, it's important to define what "winning" means to you. This is about identifying what truly matters—your core values, goals, and vision for your future.

Ask yourself:

- What are the most important areas of my life (e.g., health, career, relationships, personal growth)?
- What does success look like in each of these areas?
- What legacy do I want to create?

By clarifying your vision, you give yourself a clear target to aim for and a framework for decision-making.

2. Creating a Life Mission Statement

Your mission statement is a short, guiding principle that reflects your core purpose. It can provide direction when you face difficult choices or feel overwhelmed by competing priorities.

To create your mission statement, reflect on these prompts:

- What motivates and inspires me?
- How do I want to make a positive impact on the world?
- What strengths and passions define who I am?

For example, your mission might be:

"To lead a balanced life of growth, creativity, and service by empowering others and continuously challenging myself to improve."

Keep your mission statement visible and revisit it regularly.

3. Setting SMART Goals

Goals give you a roadmap for achieving your vision. To be effective, goals should be **SMART**:

- **Specific**: Clearly define what you want to achieve.

- **Measurable**: Set criteria to track your progress.
- **Achievable**: Ensure the goal is realistic given your current resources and constraints.
- **Relevant**: Align the goal with your broader life mission.
- **Time-bound**: Set a deadline to create urgency.

For example, instead of saying, *"I want to be healthier,"* a SMART goal would be:

"I will exercise for 30 minutes, three times a week, for the next two months."

4. Developing Daily and Weekly Rituals

Consistency is key to long-term success. Rituals help you stay grounded and focused by creating structure in your day.

Here are examples of powerful rituals:

- **Morning routine**: Start your day with meditation, journaling, or visualization to set a positive tone.
- **Workday reflection**: Take five minutes at the end of each day to review your accomplishments and plan for tomorrow.
- **Weekly check-in**: Set aside time to assess your progress toward your goals and adjust your plans if necessary.

These rituals create momentum and help you stay aligned with your priorities.

5. Managing Your Energy, Not Just Your Time

Productivity isn't just about managing time—it's also about

managing your energy. When you align tasks with your natural energy levels, you can accomplish more with less effort.

Tips for energy management:

- **Identify your peak hours**: Schedule your most demanding tasks during your peak energy periods.
- **Take regular breaks**: Use techniques like the Pomodoro method to maintain focus and prevent burnout.
- **Prioritize recovery**: Ensure you get enough sleep, exercise, and downtime to recharge.

By optimizing your energy, you can work smarter, not harder.

6. Building Mental Resilience for Setbacks

No matter how well you plan, setbacks are inevitable. Resilience is what allows you to recover quickly and keep moving forward.

To build resilience, practice the following:

- **Reframe setbacks**: View failures as learning opportunities rather than permanent defeats.
- **Focus on what you can control**: Let go of things outside your influence and take action on what you can change.
- **Seek support**: Reach out to mentors, friends, or colleagues for guidance and encouragement.

Resilience is a skill that grows with experience and reflection.

7. Mastering Focus in a Distracted World

In today's digital world, staying focused can be a challenge. To protect your attention, you need a strategy for managing distractions.

Try these focus-enhancing techniques:

- **Time-blocking**: Allocate specific periods for focused work, with no interruptions.
- **Digital detox**: Turn off notifications and set boundaries for screen time.
- **Mindfulness practices**: Regular meditation can train your brain to stay present and resist distractions.

Developing strong focus habits helps you make consistent progress toward your goals.

8. Strengthening Your Support Network

Success is rarely a solo journey. Having a strong support network can provide encouragement, accountability, and fresh perspectives.

To build and maintain your network:

- **Cultivate meaningful relationships**: Invest time in people who inspire, challenge, and support you.
- **Seek mentors**: Learn from people who have achieved what you aspire to.
- **Give back**: Support others in their goals by sharing your knowledge and resources.

Surrounding yourself with positive influences accelerates your personal and professional growth.

9. Practicing Self-Compassion and Self-Care

Achieving your goals doesn't mean pushing yourself to exhaustion. Self-compassion and self-care are essential for maintaining long-term well-being.

Ways to practice self-compassion:

- **Be kind to yourself**: Speak to yourself with the same empathy you'd offer a friend.
- **Acknowledge your progress**: Celebrate small wins and recognize your efforts.
- **Allow rest**: Schedule time for rest and relaxation without guilt.

Taking care of yourself ensures you have the mental and physical energy to pursue your ambitions.

10. Tracking Progress and Adjusting Your Course

Regular progress tracking helps you stay motivated and identify areas for improvement. Use tools like journals, habit trackers, or apps to monitor your achievements.

Questions to ask during progress reviews:

- What wins have I achieved recently?
- What challenges have I faced, and how did I respond?
- What adjustments do I need to make to stay on track?

By reflecting regularly, you can refine your strategies and stay aligned with your long-term vision.

11. Cultivating a Mindset of Lifelong Growth

Success isn't a destination—it's an ongoing journey of learning and growth. Embrace a mindset of curiosity and adaptability by:

- **Seeking new challenges**: Push yourself to learn new skills and explore unfamiliar opportunities.
- **Embracing feedback**: View constructive criticism as a tool for growth.
- **Staying curious**: Ask questions, read widely, and engage with diverse perspectives.

Lifelong growth ensures that you continue evolving in both your personal and professional life.

12. Living with Purpose and Joy

Ultimately, winning at life means living with purpose, joy, and a sense of fulfillment. It's about aligning your actions with your values, nurturing meaningful relationships, and finding gratitude in the present moment.

To live with purpose:

- **Regularly revisit your mission**: Ensure your goals and routines reflect your core values.
- **Practice gratitude**: Celebrate the journey, not just the destination.
- **Be present**: Focus on the here and now, fully experiencing each moment.

By following your mental playbook, you can navigate life's

challenges with confidence, resilience, and clarity.